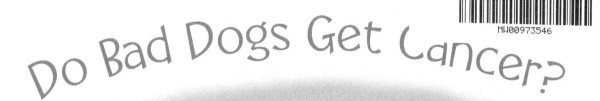

Do Bad Dogs Get Cancer?

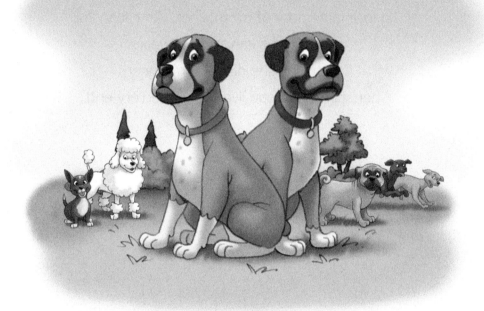

Patricia A. Brill, PhD

Illustrated by Curt Walstead

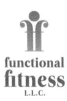

functional fitness
L.L.C.

Dedication

In loving memory of my mother, Mary Jean Brill.
She fought cancer for 9 years.
Although she died from cancer,
her spirit and hope lived until the very end.

Hello All—

The story you are about to read is about my best friend Turbo. One day while Turbo was sitting on a cold shiny bed, Dr. Larry the Vet noticed Turbo had moles on his legs and stomach. After several tests, Turbo was diagnosed with cancer. We didn't know what would happen next, but from that point on I knew I needed to be there for Turbo; to support him; and help him get through this scary ordeal.

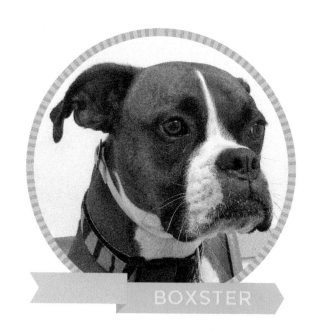

BOXSTER

It is my hope that this book will help you understand what happens after a loved one, including your pet, is diagnosed with cancer. This book will explain what cancer is, and that cancer is not contagious. Just as Turbo needed me to be there for him while he was sick; you will find that people you know who develop cancer will need you even more to be there for them.

Remember, you might not know what words to say to someone with cancer, but sometimes all they might need is a hug.

Love,

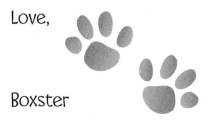

Boxster

P.S. Turbo still gets a "Bad Dog" once in a while. He can't help it.

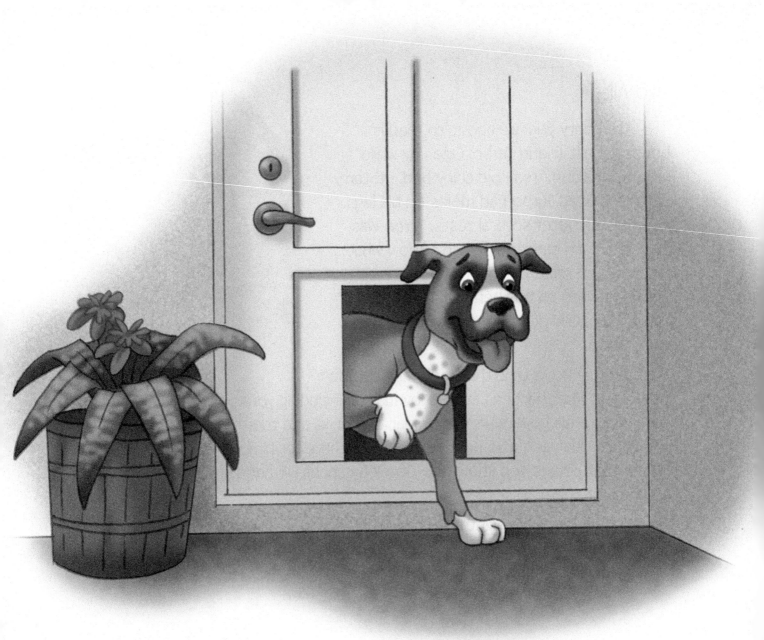

Boxster bolted through the doggie door. "Turbo" shrieked
Boxster, "the ducks are back! Let's go chase them!"

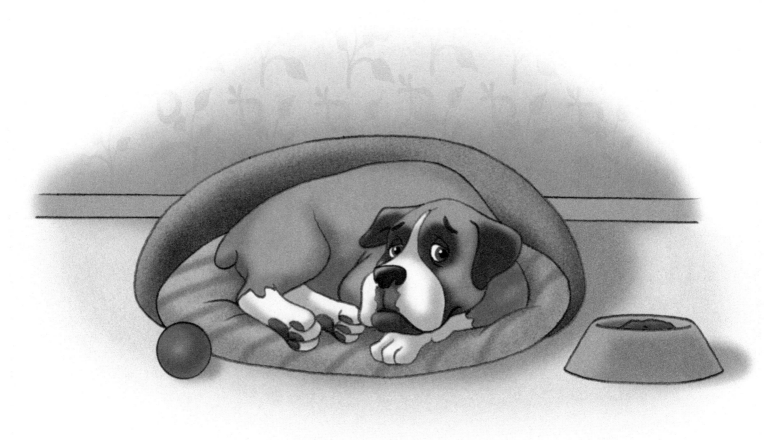

Turbo was curled up in his doggie bed, tight as a ball. His ear perked up a little but he just laid there. "I don't feel very well" Turbo sighed. "I'm too tired. I don't want to play today."

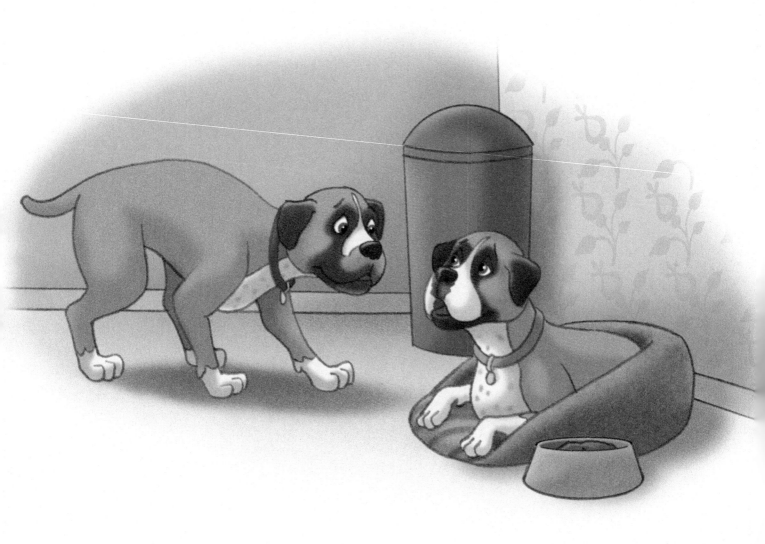

"What's wrong, Turb?" asked Boxster. "I don't know" sighed
Turbo. "I'm not hungry, and I just don't have any energy."

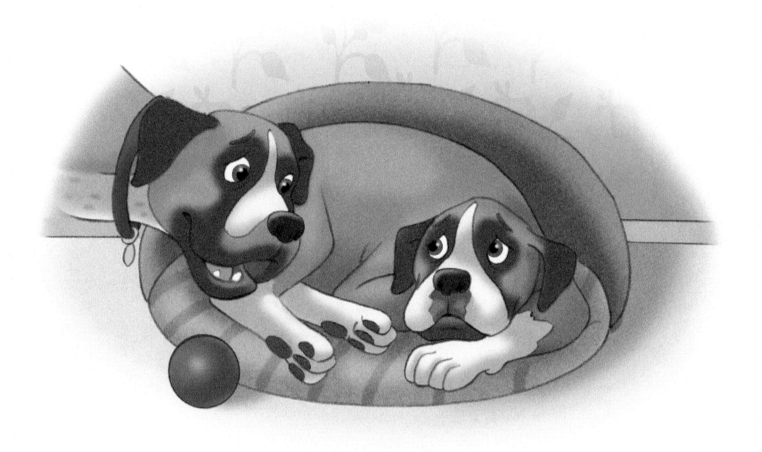

"What! Not Hungry? Something must be wrong with you!" exclaimed Boxster. "Don't worry, Turb, we'll go see Dr. Larry the Vet. He'll help you feel better."

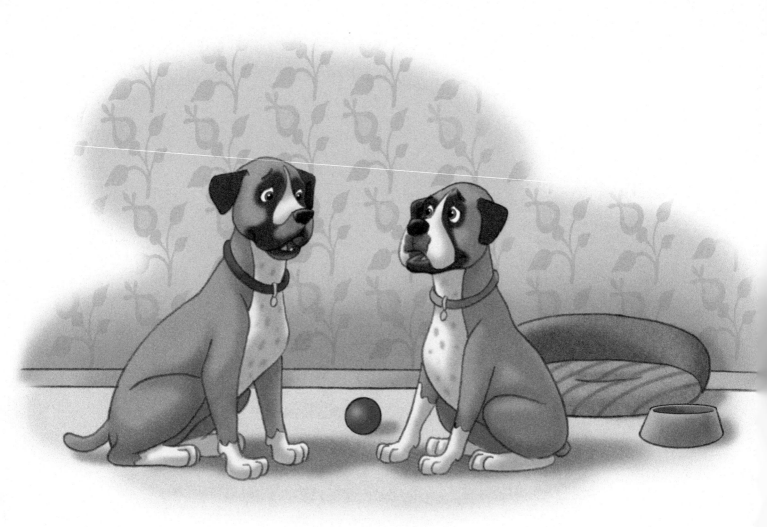

"Why do I have to go to see Dr. Larry?" asked Turbo.

"So he can run some tests to find out what's wrong with you" replied Boxster.

"Tests," whimpered Turbo. "What tests? I'm afraid of tests. Will the tests hurt?"

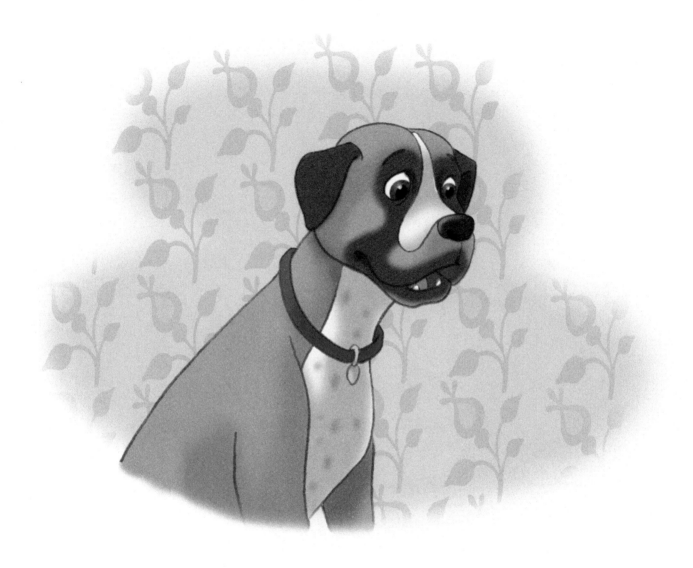

"Don't worry" assured Boxster, the tests won't hurt. However Dr. Larry the vet may have to use a needle to draw blood from you. But, it will only sting for a minute."

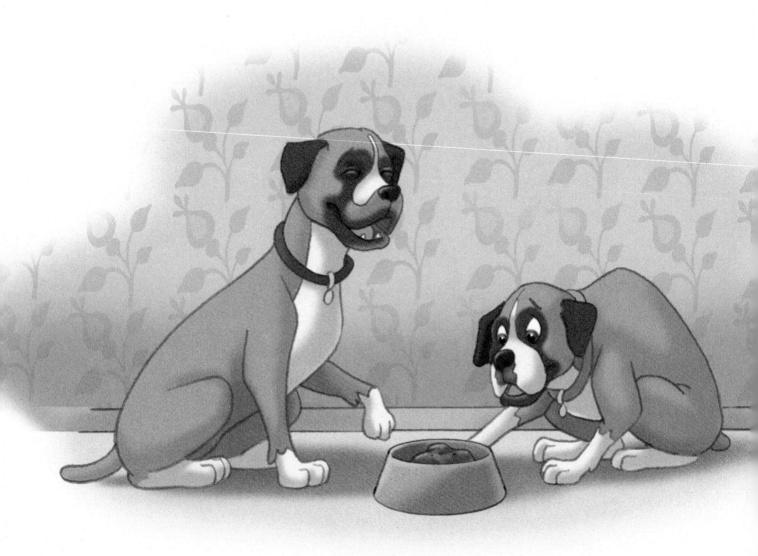

"How long is a minute?" asked Turbo. "A minute is about as long as it takes you to eat your bowl of dog food," giggled Boxster.

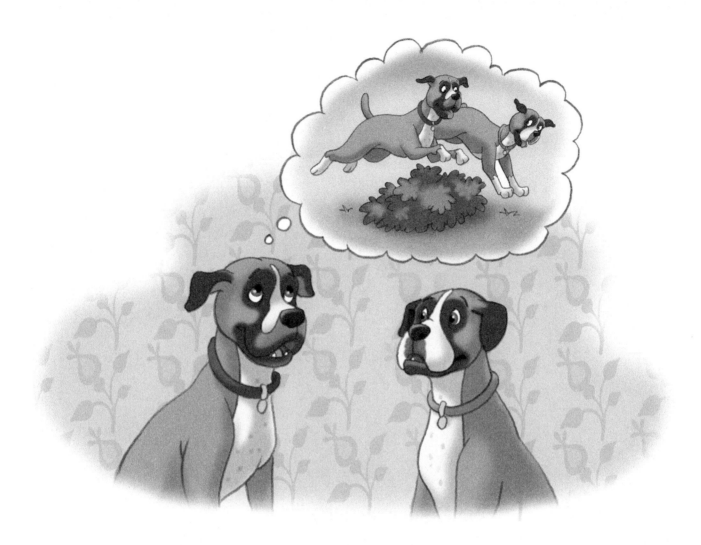

"What happens when the test results come back?" asked Turbo. Boxster replied, "The test results will tell Dr. Larry if there is something wrong with you, and if there is, he will decide what treatment you need to help you feel better. Once you are better, we can run and jump and spin and play in our big back yard without you getting so tired."

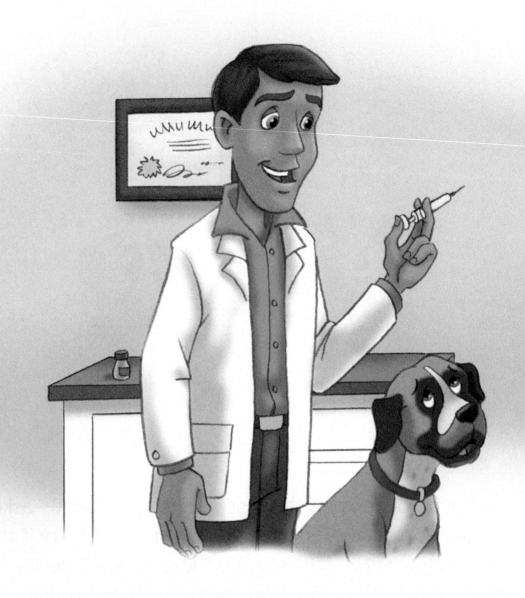

Dr. Larry lifted Turbo onto the shiny cold bed. He took Turbo's temperature and ran several tests.

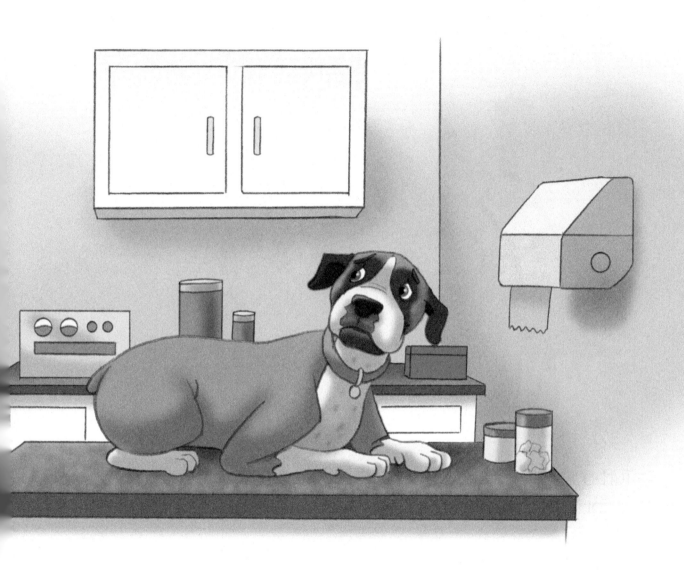

Then he poked Turbo with a needle. Turbo cocked his head to the side, "That didn't hurt at all." Dr. Larry left the room.

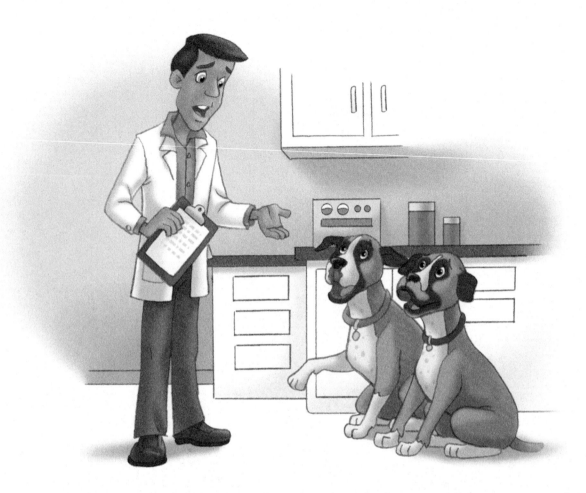

Turbo and Boxster sat pressed tightly together, patiently waiting for Dr. Larry to come back. Their hearts were pounding in their chests.

Finally Dr. Larry walked in. "I have good news and I have bad news," he said. "The bad news is that Turbo has some moles on his legs and stomach that are cancerous. "CANCER!" shrieked Turbo and Boxster.

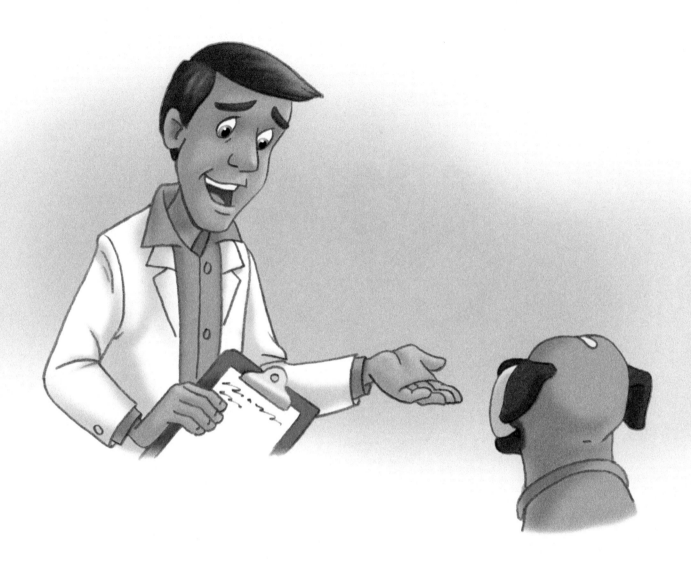

However, the good news is that the cancer is in Stage I. Turbo will have to undergo surgery to have the moles removed. And hopefully after removing the moles and undergoing treatment, the cancer will be gone."

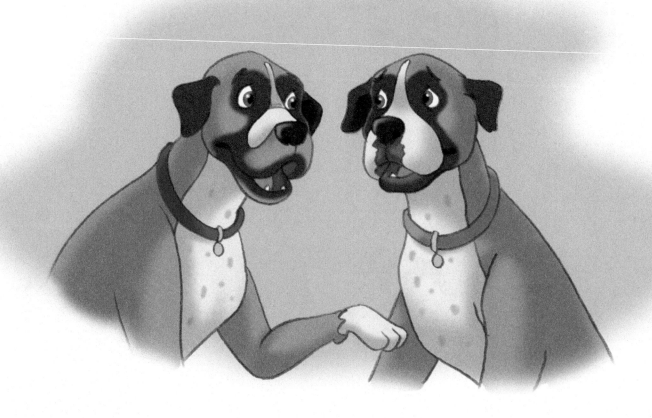

"Boxster, I'm afraid" whispered Turbo. Boxster whispered back. "Don't worry Turb. I'll help you get through this." "How can you help me?" asked Turbo. "Did you ever have cancer?"

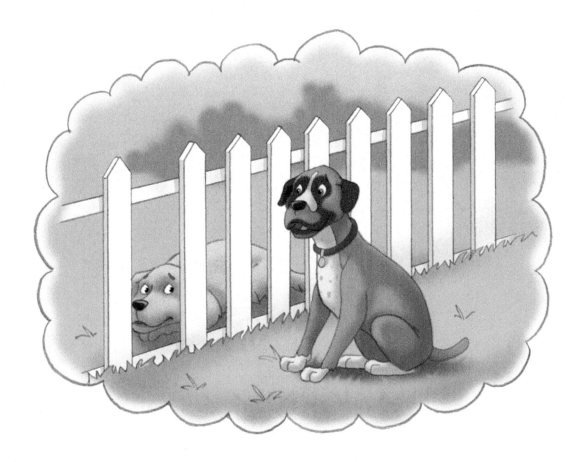

"No, I never had cancer" said Boxster. But the dog that lived next door to me named Carrera had cancer. While Carrera was sick, I would sit on the other side of the fence and talk to her because she had no one else to talk to. She would tell me how she felt, if she was tired, if she was sick to her stomach, or even if she was having a good day. So I know a little bit about what dogs go through when they have cancer."

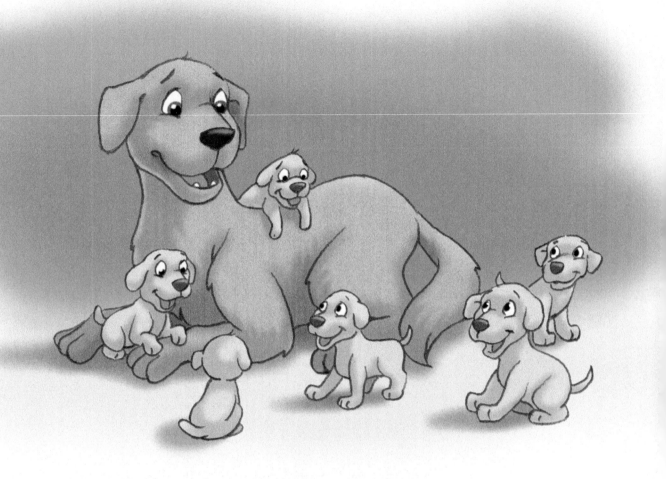

"What happened to Carrera?" asked Turbo. "Did her cancer go away?" Boxster replied. "Yes, it did, but it took her a long time to recover from the surgery and all the medications she had to take. But once her cancer was gone she had six puppies!"

"Boxster, did I get cancer because I'm being punished for being a bad dog?" cried Turbo. "No Turb" comforted Boxster. "Bad dogs get time-outs, not cancer. All types of dogs can get cancer. They might not be Boxers like us. They could be Labs, Poodles, Chihuahuas, or even Pugs. They could be black dogs or white dogs, spotted dogs, or furry dogs. They could even be fat dogs like you." "I'm not fat!" cried Turbo. "I am just big boned!"

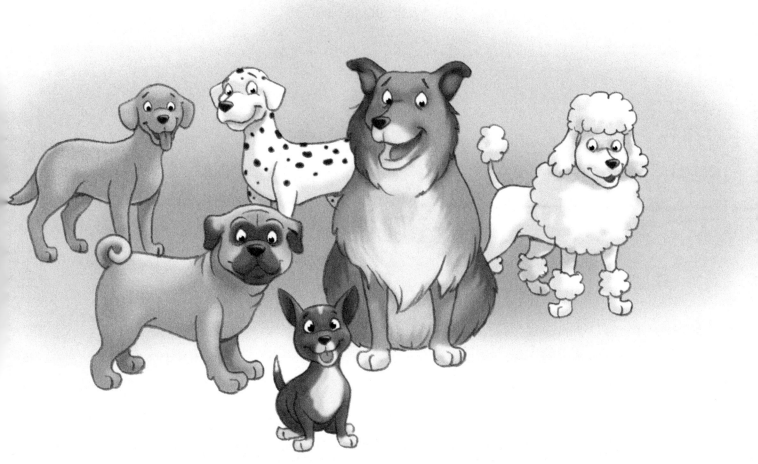

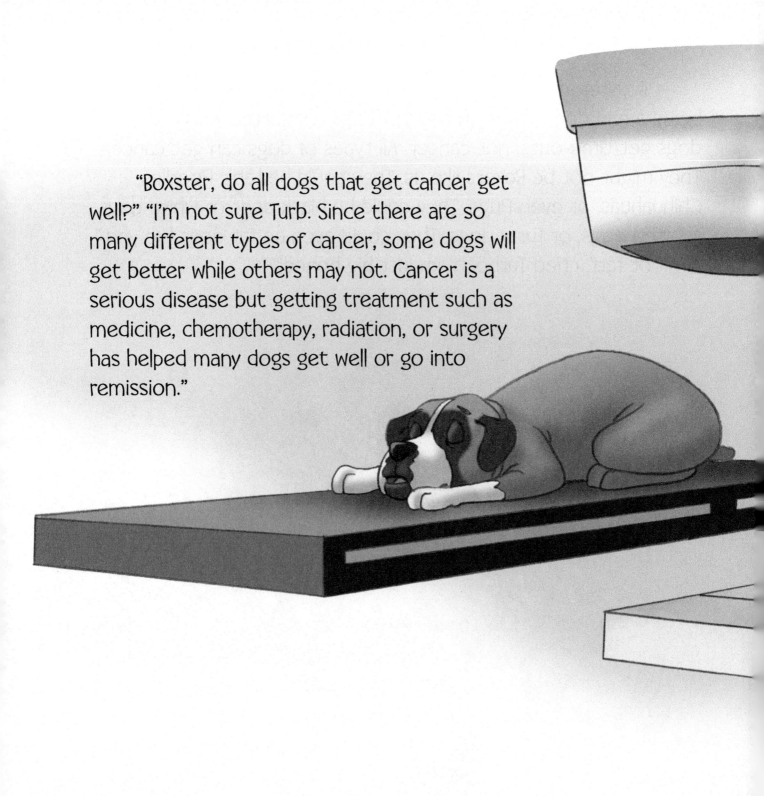

"Boxster, do all dogs that get cancer get well?" "I'm not sure Turb. Since there are so many different types of cancer, some dogs will get better while others may not. Cancer is a serious disease but getting treatment such as medicine, chemotherapy, radiation, or surgery has helped many dogs get well or go into remission."

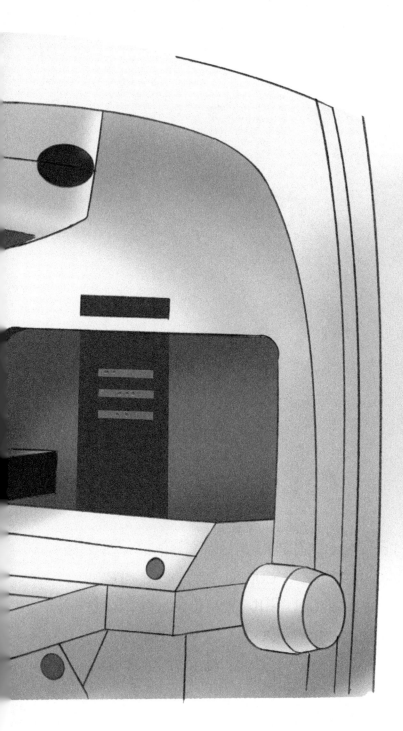

"Those big words sound scary" said Turbo. "What do they mean?" Boxster replied. "Chemotherapy and radiation are keys to fighting cancer. They are different treatments Dr. Larry might give you as a way to help your sick cells get better."

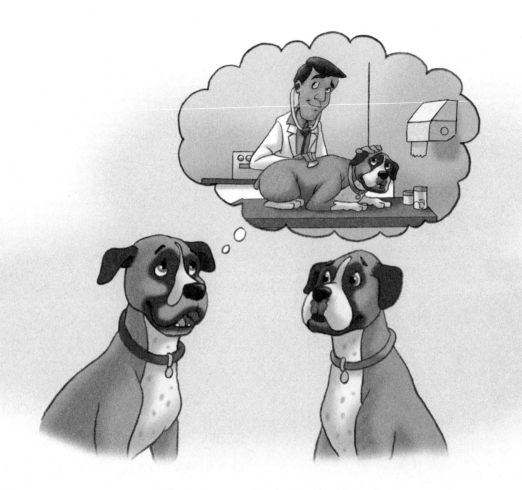

"What is remission, Boxster?" asked Turbo.

"Remission is when the cancer may be cured or there are no more signs or symptoms of the cancer. But don't worry, Turb" assured Boxster, once you are in remission, Dr. Larry will run tests and monitor you closely to make sure the cancer doesn't come back."

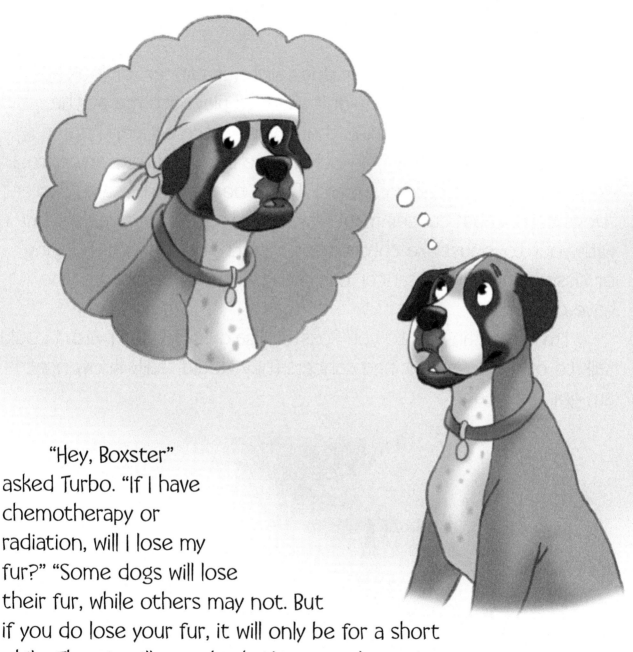

"Hey, Boxster"
asked Turbo. "If I have
chemotherapy or
radiation, will I lose my
fur?" "Some dogs will lose
their fur, while others may not. But
if you do lose your fur, it will only be for a short
while. Then it will grow back. Most people won't
even notice. Hey, you could wear a bandana!"

Turbo sighed. "Now other dogs without cancer will look at me like I am different. They won't want to play with me at the dog park because they'll think they might catch cancer. I don't think we should even sleep in our doggie bed together anymore. I don't want you to catch cancer." "Don't be silly, Turb" said Boxster." "Dogs can't catch cancer from playing with other dogs or playing with your toys; just like children can't catch cancer from hugging or kissing adults with cancer or playing with other children who have cancer."

I'm glad I can talk to you Boxster," said Turbo. But I wish I could talk to other dogs that had cancer. They would really know what I am going through."

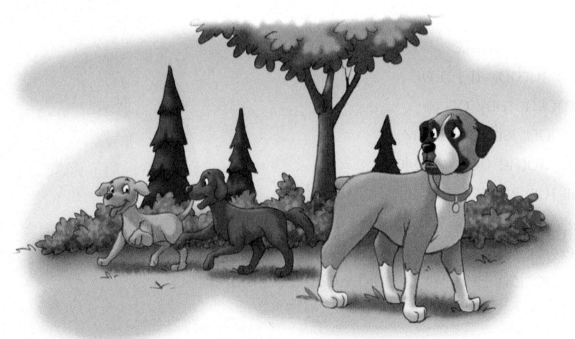

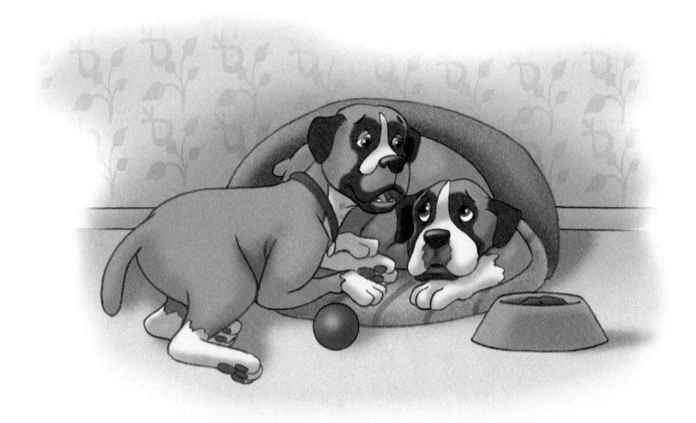

Exhausted by the stress of the day, and worried about his upcoming surgery, Turbo circled three times then curled up in his doggie bed. Boxster snuggled tight next to him. "I'm scared," whimpered Turbo. "But if you stay with me then I know I will be brave." Boxster replied "It's Okay to be scared, Turb. Remember, you are not alone in this struggle. If you are ever scared or sad, angry or mad you can always come and talk to me. I will always be there for you. Remember we will be best friends forever!"

The next day Turbo underwent surgery to have his moles removed. Boxster waited patiently for Turbo to get out of the operating room. Finally Turbo came back into the small room.

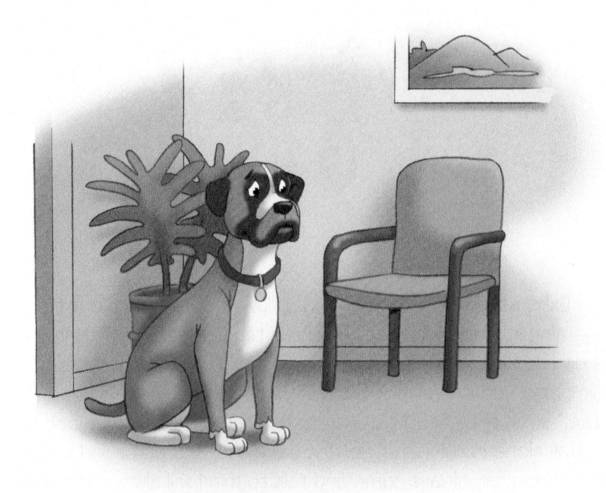

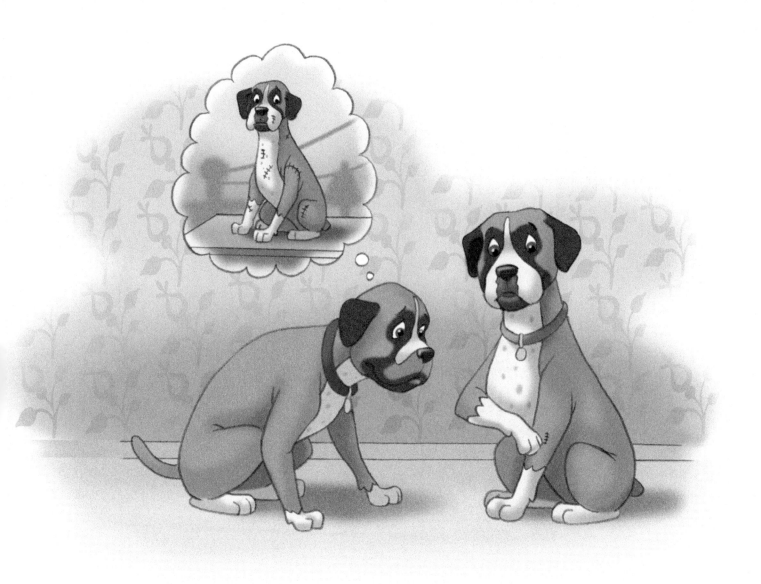

"Boxster look!" cried Turbo. "Dr. Larry shaved my fur to remove my cancerous moles. I have stitches all over my body." "Don't worry Turbo" said Boxster. "This year for Halloween you can go as Frankendog!"

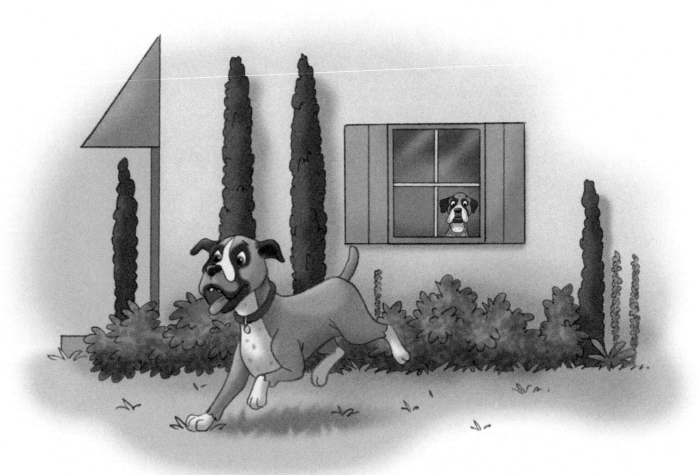

As the weeks went by, Turbo would sit in the window and watch Boxster play. "Boxster," asked Turbo, "what did you do today? Did you catch a squirrel? Did you dash around the back yard? Did you run and jump and spin and play?"

"I didn't do anything fun today," muttered Boxster.

"Boxster, you can tell me about your day" assured Turbo. "Although I don't feel like spinning and jumping and playing with my toys yet, I still want to hear about the fun you had. Knowing that you did something fun doesn't make me sad. It makes me feel better. If you want, you can even play with my toys." "WHAT!" exclaimed Boxster? "You never share your toys." Turbo's stub of a tail slowly wagged.

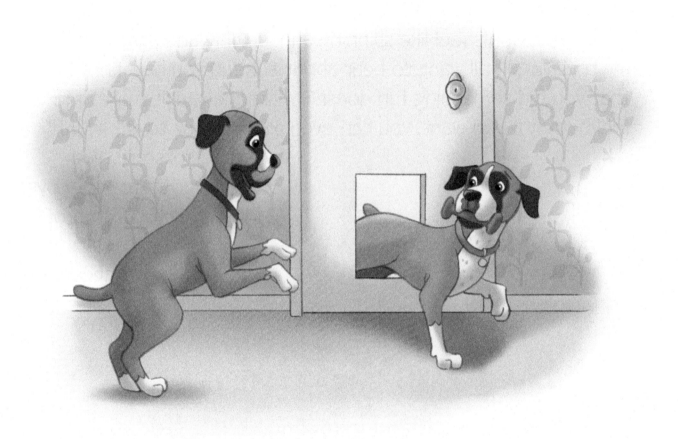

Finally one day Turbo darted out the doggie door then ran back inside with his favorite toy. "Turb!" shouted Boxster. "You must be feeling better. You've got a toy – Hurray!"

That night before they fell asleep in their doggie bed, Turbo said to Boxster, "Boxster, now I know I didn't get cancer because I was being punished for being a bad dog. So I hope other dogs will realize that as well.

Thanks for being with me through all of this." "You're welcome Turb," said Boxster. "That's what best friends are for."

"Good Night Turbo,"
"Good Night Boxster"
"We'll have more fun tomorrow!"

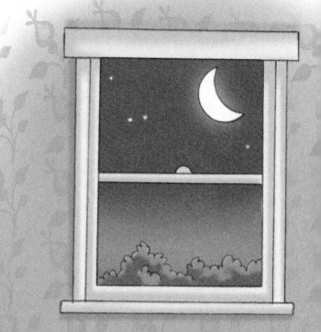

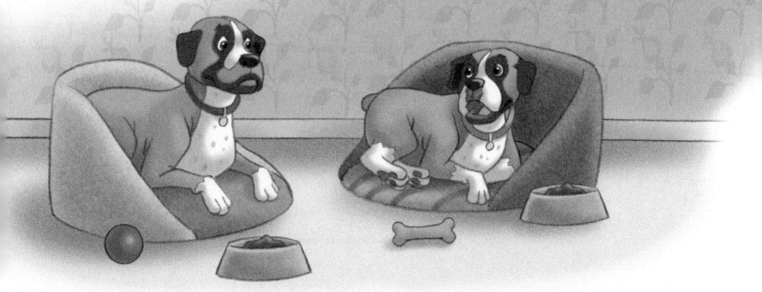

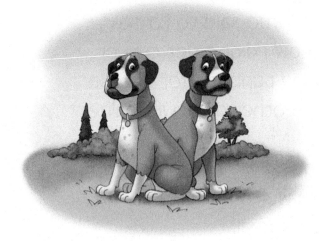

∽

CPSIA information can be obtained
at www.ICGtesting.com
Printed in the USA
LVOW02s1051270516

489632LV00040B/33/P